Dr. Adrian Selby

FREE YOURSELF FROM GRAPHENE

The Ultimate Solution to Detoxify Your Body

"The human body is the best picture of the soul."

– Ludwig Wittgenstein

Index

1. Introduction

2. Understanding Graphene: A Revolutionary Material

- What is Graphene?

- Unique Properties of Graphene

- Technological and Medical Applications

3. Promises and Risks of Nanotechnology

- Controversies about Graphene and Health Concerns

4. The Effects of Graphene on the Human Body

- Biological Effects of Graphene

- Accumulation in Vital Organs: Liver, Kidneys, Lungs, and Brain

- Long-Term Effects and Need for Further Studies

5. How to Detect Graphene in the Body

- Raman Spectroscopy

- Electron Microscopy (SEM and TEM)

- Emerging Biosensors and Mass Spectrometry Technique

6. The Body's Natural Detoxification Mechanisms

- Role of the Immune System
- Detoxification Processes in the Liver and Kidneys
- Lymphatic Drainage and Excretion Pathways

7. Natural Strategies for Detoxifying from Graphene

- Antioxidant-Rich Diets
- Key Supplements: Glutathione, NAC, Milk Thistle, and Zeolite
- Hydration, Physical Activity, and Detoxifying Teas
- Breathing Techniques and Sauna Therapy

8. Success Stories and Testimonials

- Real-Life Detoxification Journeys
- Case Studies of Health Improvements

9. The Evolving Research on Graphene

- Recent Discoveries on Graphene's Biological Effects
- Innovations in Nanomedicine
- Mechanisms of Graphene Elimination and Future Therapies

10. Tools for Health Monitoring and Home Evaluation

- Wearable Devices and Biosensors
- Self-Assessment Kits for Oxidative Stress and Toxin Levels
- Home Practices for Reducing Toxins

11. Future Innovations and Potential Drugs for Graphene

- Emerging Therapies: Enzymatic Nanoparticles and Nanocapsules
- Personalized Detoxification Strategies
- Advancements in Monitoring Technologies

12. Final Reflections

- Key Takeaways on Graphene and Health
- Integrating Natural and Technological Solutions
- Preparing for a Safer Future

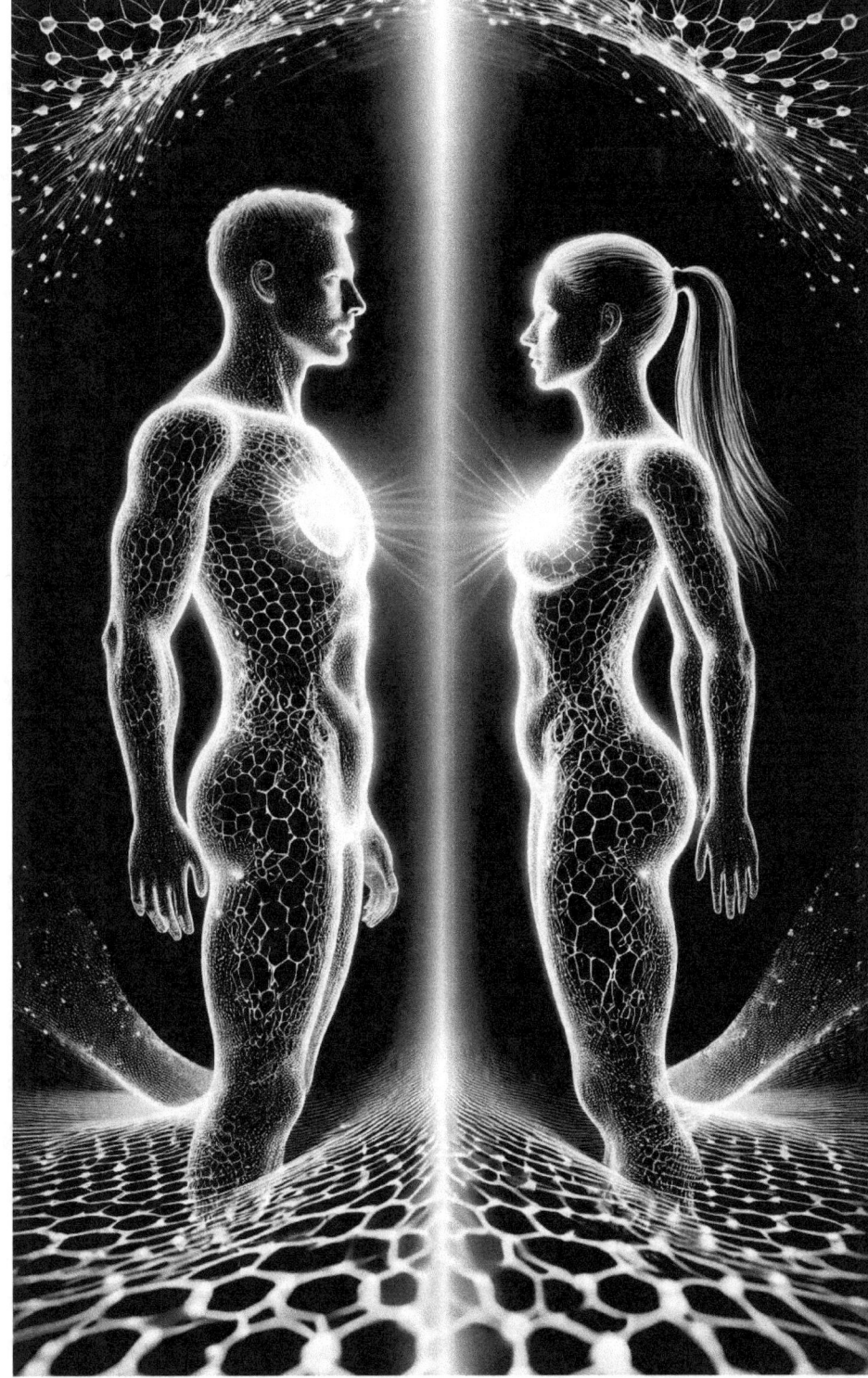

Introduction

The advent of nanotechnology has unlocked new frontiers in material science, offering extraordinary solutions across various fields, from medicine to energy, technology, and construction. However, with the introduction of innovative materials like graphene, new challenges arise, particularly regarding their safety and impact on human health.

Graphene - a light and ultra-thin material - is often hailed as the "wonder material" due to its exceptional properties, such as electrical conductivity, mechanical strength, and flexibility. Despite its revolutionary potential, many questions remain about the long-term effects of prolonged exposure to graphene, especially in environments where it could enter the body in the form of nanoparticles.

This guide delves into the complex relationship between graphene and human health, aiming to answer some of the most pressing questions about how our bodies react to exposure to this material. Through the analysis of recent studies and natural detoxification strategies, we offer practical pathways to safeguard our health and mitigate the potential risks associated with this new technology.

By the end, readers will have a clearer understanding of how to balance the benefits of technological advancement with proactive steps to protect their well-being in an increasingly nanomaterial-driven world.

For over two decades, I have dedicated my career to studying the impact of nanoparticles on the human body, with a special focus on the novel materials increasingly entering our daily environment. My work was born from the belief that every innovation, no matter how promising, must be thoroughly evaluated and understood in terms of its risks as well as its benefits.

Graphene is, without a doubt, one of the most fascinating discoveries of our time. Its applications seem endless: from flexible electronics circuits to medical diagnostic sensors, from solar cells to energy storage technologies. However, its growing usage has highlighted a less discussed aspect: the effects of graphene on human health.

This guide you hold in your hands stems from my personal commitment to raising greater awareness on this subject. In a world increasingly reliant on nanotechnology, it is crucial to understand the potential risks and take preventive measures to protect our bodies.

Throughout my career, I have witnessed how science can improve people's lives, but I have also seen the risks associated with the unregulated introduction of new technologies. Graphene, despite its extraordinary qualities, is not exempt from these risks. As a researcher, I feel it is my duty to share with you the knowledge you need to navigate this new technological landscape safely.

I hope this guide not only equips you with the tools to better understand the impact of graphene but also inspires you to take an active role in your health and the monitoring of this remarkable and complex material.

Preface: Dr. Adrian Selby, PhD
Independent Researcher in Nanotechnology and Biomedical Safety

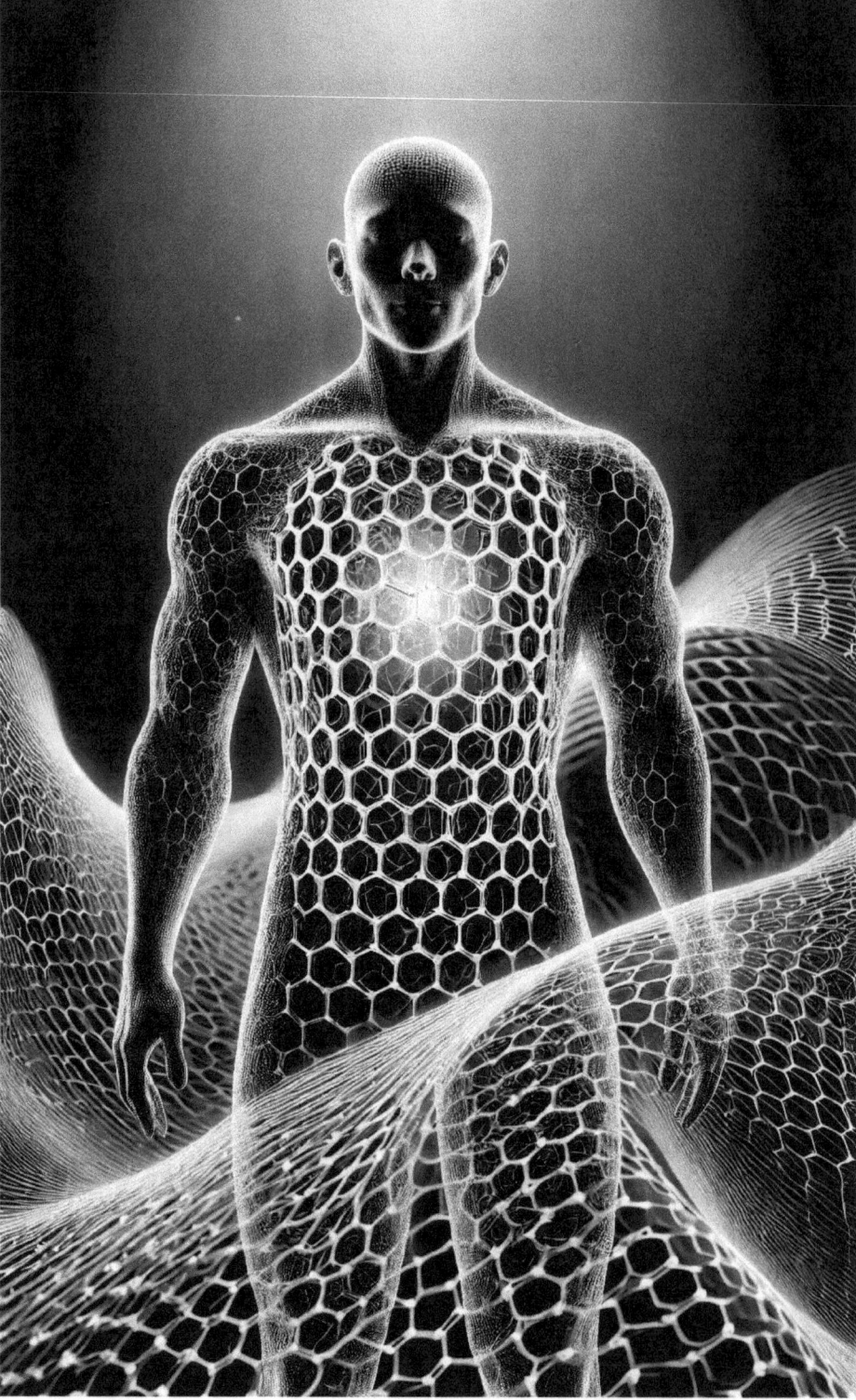

Chapter 1: What is Graphene?

Graphene is one of the most extraordinary materials ever discovered. Composed of a single layer of carbon atoms arranged in a honeycomb lattice, it is considered the thinnest material in existence. Its discovery, awarded the Nobel Prize in Physics in 2010, opened new pathways in scientific research and technological innovation. Graphene boasts exceptional properties: it is about 200 times stronger than steel, yet it is also extremely flexible, lightweight, and nearly transparent. Additionally, it is an excellent conductor of both heat and electricity, making it useful for a wide range of applications, from the technology sector to biomedical uses.

Unique Properties of Graphene

One of the most fascinating aspects of graphene is its electrical conductivity. Because electrons move extraordinarily fast through its two-dimensional structure, graphene can be used as a key component to create faster and more efficient electronic circuits than traditional materials like silicon. This characteristic makes it an ideal candidate for the next generation of electronic devices, such as smartphones, tablets, batteries, and superconductors.

Additionally, graphene has high thermal conductivity, meaning it can dissipate heat extremely efficiently. This makes it valuable in technologies that require rapid heat transfer, such as computer heat sinks and cooling systems.

Lastly, graphene is biocompatible, meaning it can interact with biological tissues without causing significant damage. This property makes it ideal for the development of innovative biosensors and medical devices.

Technological and Medical Applications

The technology and biomedical industries are heavily investing in the development of applications that utilize graphene. For instance:

- **Graphene batteries:** Lithium-ion batteries, commonly used in phones and laptops, could be replaced by graphene batteries. These batteries promise longer life and faster charging times. Companies like Samsung and others are working on graphene battery prototypes that could revolutionize the energy storage sector.

- **Water filtration membranes:** Graphene has the ability to efficiently filter harmful substances from water, such as salts and pathogens, making it a potential solution for improving access to clean drinking water globally.

- **Medical devices and biosensors:** Thanks to its conductivity and biocompatibility, graphene is being studied for the development of biosensors that can monitor physiological parameters in real time, such as blood glucose levels, or detect diseases with high precision.

Controversies about Graphene and Health Concerns

Despite its revolutionary potential, graphene is also at the center of various controversies, particularly concerning its possible presence in vaccines and related health concerns.

Presence in vaccines: Some activist groups have raised concerns about the alleged presence of graphene in COVID-19 vaccines, suggesting that graphene oxide nanoparticles could be used as adjuvants or drug carriers. However, there is no scientific evidence to support these claims. Studies on COVID-19 vaccines do not indicate the presence of graphene or its derivatives among the ingredients approved by regulatory agencies, such as the EMA and FDA. Nonetheless, the widespread circulation of these rumors has raised questions about the safety of graphene in the human body.

Health effects: Graphene is a relatively new material, and its effects on the human body are still under study. Some research suggests that prolonged inhalation of graphene nanoparticles could have toxic effects, particularly in the lungs, leading to inflammation and tissue damage. Preclinical studies conducted on animal models have shown that graphene may cause oxidative stress, a process that damages cells due to the buildup of free radicals. While there is no evidence that graphene is dangerous to human health under normal usage conditions, further work is needed to better understand how the human body reacts to prolonged exposure to this material.

Research on Graphene's Biological Effects

Several studies have examined how graphene interacts with biological tissues. An experiment published in ACS Nano showed that while graphene is biocompatible in controlled doses, exposure to higher amounts could impair immune cell function. This raised questions about the safety of graphene nanoparticles when used in medical or industrial contexts.

Regulating Graphene

Due to emerging concerns about the safety of graphene, regulatory agencies are considering stricter regulations for its use, particularly in medical applications. Leading health agencies such as the **World Health Organization (WHO) and the European Commission for Nanomaterials** are monitoring the situation and promoting further studies on graphene's toxicity.
Current research suggests that graphene can be used safely but requires caution when applied in ways that could lead to direct exposure to the human body, such as in implantable medical devices or pharmaceuticals.

Conclusion

Graphene represents one of the most significant discoveries in recent decades, with applications ranging from medical technology to sustainable energy. However, as with all innovations, it is crucial to consider the possible risks to human health and the environment. While there is not yet enough evidence to declare graphene dangerous, more studies are necessary to fully understand its effects on the human body, especially in terms of long-term exposure.

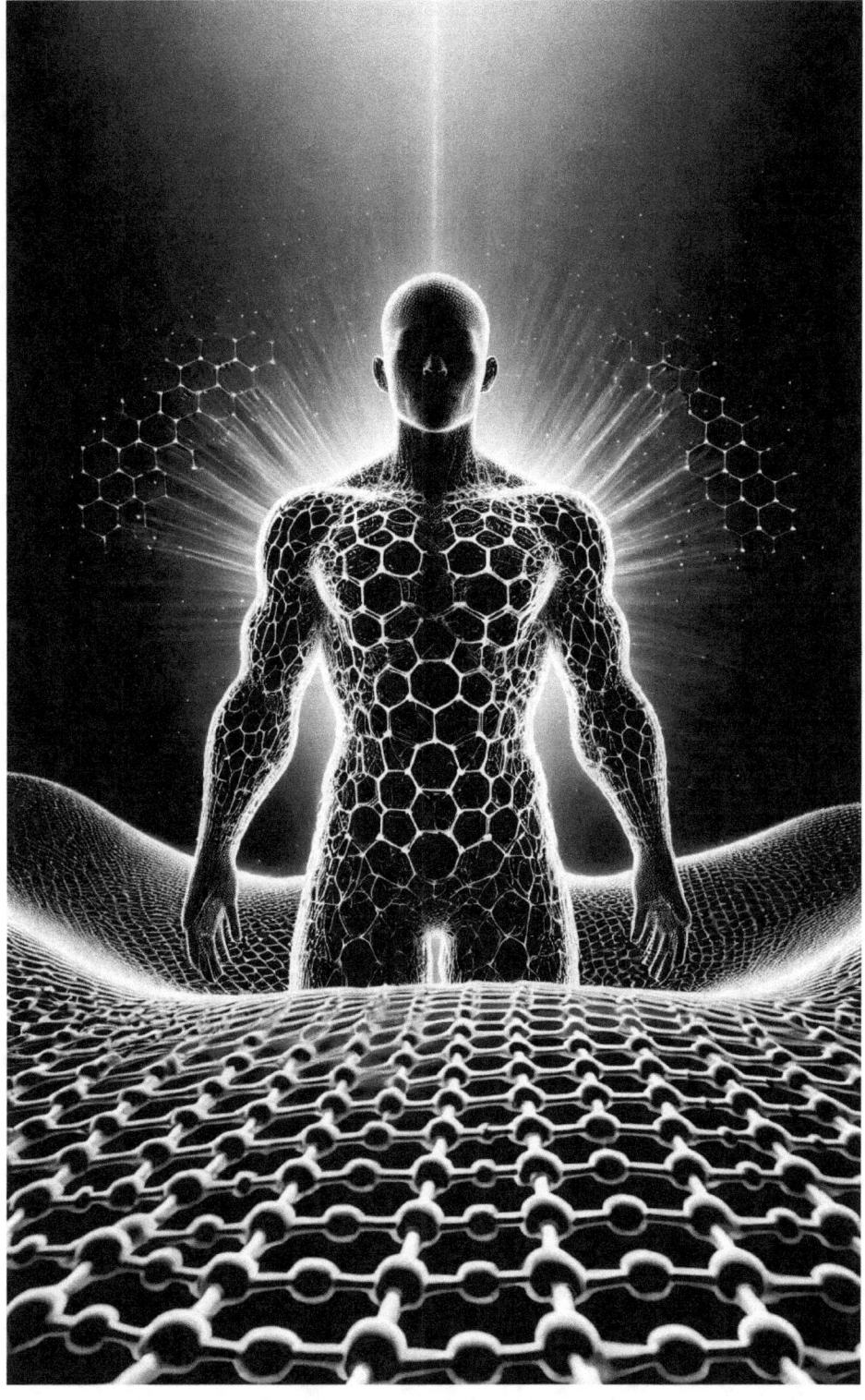

Chapter 2: The Effects of Graphene on the Human Body

Graphene's interaction with the human body, particularly its effects on vital organs, has been a topic of growing scientific interest. As a relatively new material, the long-term effects of exposure to graphene nanoparticles are still under study. Some research suggests that when inhaled or introduced into the bloodstream, graphene could accumulate in critical organs, such as the lungs, liver, and brain, potentially leading to inflammation or tissue damage.

1. Biological Effects of Graphene

Graphene nanoparticles, such as graphene oxide, can interact with cells in complex ways. Several studies indicate that these nanoparticles can cause oxidative stress, a harmful condition that disrupts normal cellular function.

Oxidative and Inflammatory Stress

Oxidative stress is one of the primary mechanisms of cellular damage caused by graphene nanoparticles. When in contact with cells, graphene nanoparticles can trigger the production of reactive oxygen species (ROS), unstable molecules that damage proteins, lipids, and DNA. A study published in *Environmental Science & Technology* showed that cells exposed to graphene oxide experienced significant oxidative damage.

Chronic inflammation is particularly concerning because it can contribute to the development of degenerative diseases, such as cancer, and the decline of organ function.

In animal models, graphene oxide has shown pro-inflammatory effects in the respiratory system, liver, and other organs. This includes the overactivation of immune responses and the release of inflammatory cytokines, which can lead to tissue damage and impaired organ function over time.

Cytotoxicity and Genotoxicity

Some studies suggest that graphene could have cytotoxic and genotoxic effects on various types of cells. In an experiment conducted on human lung cells *(in vitro)*, exposure to graphene oxide caused apoptosis (programmed cell death) and disrupted DNA repair mechanisms. This raises concerns about possible genotoxic effects, which could contribute to cellular mutations and increase the risk of tumor development.

2. Accumulation of Graphene in Vital Organs

One of the primary concerns regarding graphene is its accumulation in vital organs, such as the liver, lungs, kidneys, and brain. This accumulation may impair the function of these organs, leading to long-term consequences.

Liver and Kidneys

The liver and kidneys play a crucial role in filtering toxins and foreign substances from the body. However, studies conducted on animals have shown that graphene nanoparticles can accumulate in these organs, causing damage. In a 2016 study published in *Nanotoxicology*, researchers found that mice exposed to high doses of graphene oxide showed increased liver inflammation and signs of kidney failure.

Graphene oxide particles can be absorbed by macrophages (immune cells responsible for phagocytosis), but this process is slow and inefficient when the particle load is high. This can lead to toxic accumulation in excretory organs, impairing their ability to filter toxins.

Lungs

Exposure to graphene nanoparticles through inhalation has been associated with severe lung damage. A study published in ACS Nano examined the effects of graphene inhalation in rats and found an inflammatory response similar to that caused by asbestos. Graphene oxide, in particular, has been linked to pulmonary fibrosis, a condition where lung tissue becomes scarred and stiff, limiting the lungs' ability to function properly.

These findings suggest that in industrial environments or conditions of prolonged exposure, inhalation of graphene particles may pose significant risks to respiratory health.

Brain and Blood-Brain Barrier

One of the most concerning aspects of graphene exposure is its ability to cross the blood-brain barrier (BBB), a protective barrier that prevents harmful substances from reaching the brain. Studies conducted on animal models have shown that graphene nanoparticles can penetrate this barrier and accumulate in the brain, with potential neurotoxic effects. This raises concerns about possible links between graphene exposure and neurodegenerative diseases, such as Alzheimer's and Parkinson's. The brain is particularly vulnerable to the effects of oxidative stress, and the accumulation of toxic particles like graphene could contribute to the deterioration of cognitive and nervous functions.

3. Biological Barriers and Nanoparticle Transport

In addition to the blood-brain barrier, other biological barriers play a crucial role in limiting the spread of toxic substances throughout the body. However, graphene has demonstrated the ability to overcome various barriers, raising concerns about its long-term effects.

Placenta and Fetal Development

One of the most delicate issues concerns the possibility that graphene could cross the placenta, exposing the fetus to potentially harmful substances. Preliminary studies conducted on animal models suggest that graphene nanoparticles can accumulate in the placenta, increasing the risk of fetal malformations and damage to the developing central nervous system. Although research is still limited, this aspect requires further investigation, especially in contexts where graphene could be used in implantable medical devices or drugs.

4. Long-Term Effects and the Need for Further Studies

Currently, most studies on the effects of graphene on the human body have been conducted on animal models or cell cultures. While these studies provide valuable insights, there is an urgent need for long-term human studies to fully understand the effects of graphene nanoparticles. The **European Commission for Nanomaterials** and other institutions are currently promoting more in-depth research to determine the safety of graphene in commercial and medical applications.

Conclusion

Graphene holds extraordinary potential, but its interactions with the human body raise complex questions. Preliminary studies suggest that exposure to graphene, particularly in the form of nanoparticles, may lead to oxidative stress, inflammation, and damage to vital organs. While these risks need to be further investigated, it is essential to remain aware of graphene's potential effects on health.

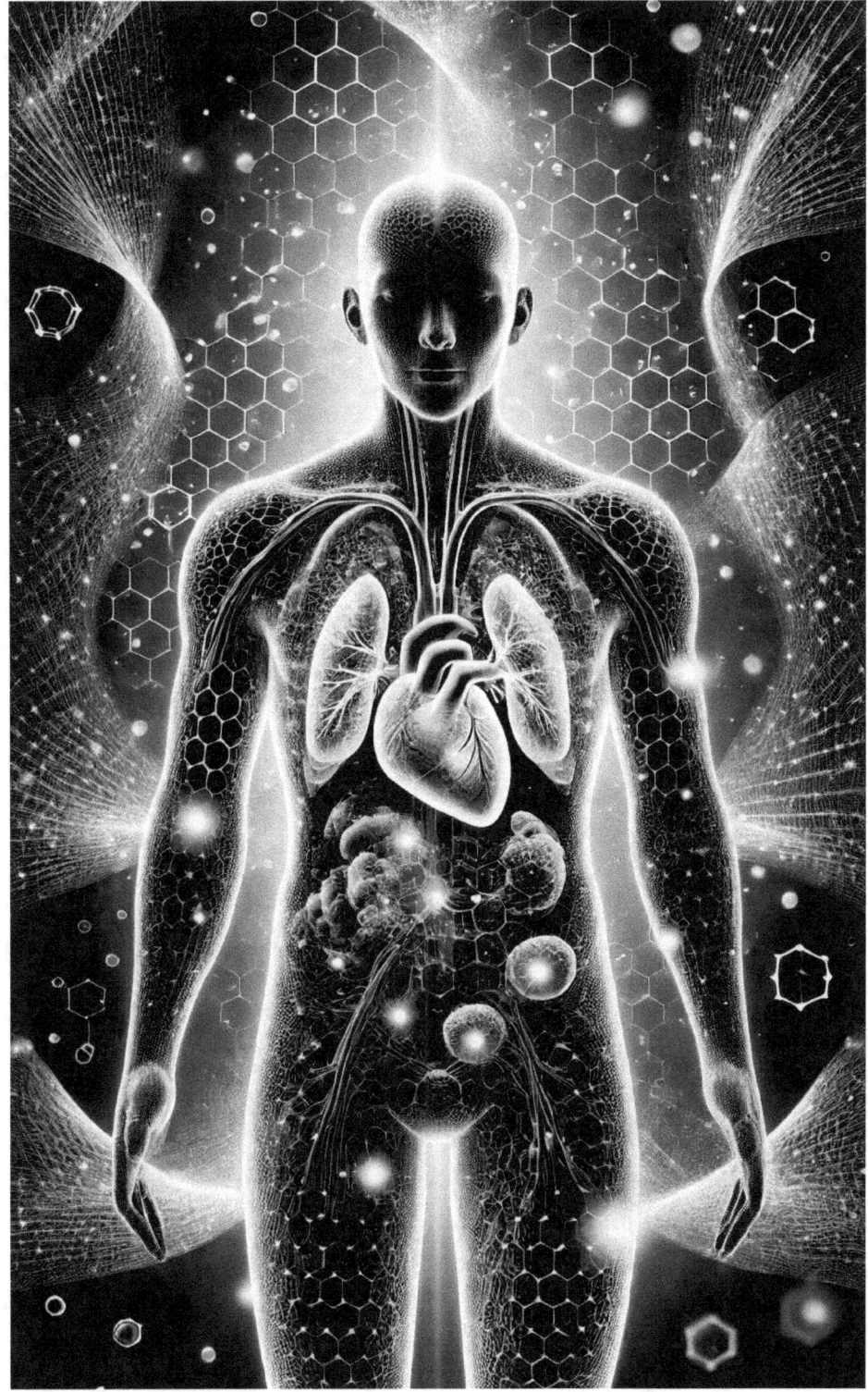

Chapter 3: How is Graphene Detected in the Body?

As discussed in previous chapters, graphene is an extremely versatile yet complex material. Despite its promising applications, concerns about its potential negative health effects have driven the scientific community to develop techniques for monitoring its presence in the human body. This chapter focuses on the current technologies used to detect graphene in the body and explains how these methods can provide crucial information for understanding the accumulation and biological effects of graphene nanoparticles.

1. Raman Spectroscopy: A Reliable Technique for Detecting Graphene

One of the most advanced techniques for detecting graphene is Raman spectroscopy, a method based on the analysis of inelastic scattering of light. When a laser light hits the material, the molecules in graphene emit distinctive signals that allow for the identification of its presence and properties.

Raman spectroscopy is considered a highly sensitive method for detecting graphene and is used in laboratories worldwide to monitor the quality and purity of the material. For instance, a study published in Nature Nanotechnology demonstrated how Raman spectroscopy can precisely identify even the smallest amounts of graphene oxide in biological samples, making it one of the most promising techniques for monitoring nanoparticles in the human body.

Use of Raman Spectroscopy in the Human Body

In the biomedical field, Raman spectroscopy has the potential to detect graphene nanoparticles in tissues and bodily fluids. Although the technique is currently used primarily in laboratory settings, researchers are developing more miniaturized and non-invasive versions that could be employed for medical monitoring.

One of the advantages of Raman spectroscopy is its ability to distinguish graphene from other carbon-based materials, such as nanotubes and soot, making it particularly useful for specifically monitoring graphene accumulation.

2. Electron Microscopy: Nanometric-Level Detection

Electron microscopy is another key technique used to detect graphene and other nanoparticles in the body. While Raman spectroscopy focuses on the optical properties of the material, electron microscopy uses beams of electrons to directly visualize nanoparticles at the nanometric level.

Scanning Electron Microscopy (SEM)

Scanning Electron Microscopy (SEM) can create extremely high-resolution images of tissue surfaces, allowing scientists to detect graphene nanoparticles with great precision. In an experiment conducted at the University of Manchester, researchers successfully identified graphene nanoparticles within the lung tissues of animals exposed to inhalation of graphene oxide. The use of electron microscopy allowed for direct observation of the particles and their behavior inside the body.

Transmission Electron Microscopy (TEM)

Transmission Electron Microscopy (TEM) allows for even deeper observation, enabling the visualization of nanoparticles within cells and the study of interactions between graphene and cellular structures. This is particularly useful for understanding how nanoparticles cross cell membranes and interact with internal organelles.

A study published in ACS Nano used TEM to observe how graphene nanoparticles were engulfed by macrophages, the immune system cells responsible for removing foreign substances from the body. The results showed that although macrophages can phagocytize graphene, excessive nanoparticle accumulation may interfere with their function, causing cellular damage.

3. Biosensors: The Future of Graphene Monitoring

In addition to traditional techniques, biosensors represent one of the most innovative areas in the detection of graphene nanoparticles. Biosensors are miniaturized devices that combine biological components with electronic technologies to detect specific molecules or particles in the body rapidly and non-invasively.

Graphene-Based Biosensors

An especially interesting development is the creation of graphene-based biosensors. Since graphene is an excellent conductor of electricity, it has been used to develop ultra-sensitive biosensors capable of detecting small amounts of biological substances, toxins, and nanoparticles.

This may seem paradoxical, but graphene's ability to interact with the body can be exploited to detect its presence through the use of biosensors.

For instance, a graphene biosensor developed at the University of California can detect extremely low concentrations of graphene nanoparticles in bodily fluids. The device uses a thin film of graphene which, when it comes into contact with target nanoparticles, generates an electrical signal that can be easily measured. Although this technology is still in the experimental phase, it represents a promising opportunity for the non-invasive monitoring of graphene in the human body.

Advantages of Biosensors

One of the primary advantages of biosensors is their non-invasiveness. Unlike Raman spectroscopy or electron microscopy, which require biological samples or complex procedures, biosensors can be integrated into wearable devices that continuously monitor the patient's health.
In the future, graphene-based biosensors could be used to:

• Detect the accumulation of graphene in the blood or tissues.

• Monitor toxin levels in the body and provide real-time feedback.

• Identify potential issues related to graphene exposure early, before they cause significant damage.

4. Mass Spectrometry Techniques for Detecting Graphene

Another emerging methodology for detecting graphene in the body is mass spectrometry, a technique that allows for the chemical analysis of materials at the molecular level. Mass spectrometry can be used to identify and quantify graphene nanoparticles in biological samples.

Inductively Coupled Plasma Mass Spectrometry (ICP-MS)

Inductively Coupled Plasma Mass Spectrometry (ICP-MS) is an advanced technique used to detect trace amounts of nanoparticles in complex samples like blood or tissues. A study published in the Journal of Analytical Chemistry demonstrated that ICP-MS can detect graphene nanoparticles at extremely low concentrations, making it an ideal technique for monitoring the accumulation of graphene in the human body.

ICP-MS could be used in the future to analyze tissue or bodily fluid samples to detect graphene nanoparticles in patients exposed to high levels of the material, allowing for precise monitoring and health risk assessment.

5. The Need for More Accessible Detection Technologies

Although the technologies discussed so far are highly advanced, many are currently only available in research laboratories. There is a growing need to develop diagnostic tools that can be more easily used in clinical settings to monitor patients at risk of graphene exposure.

Future advancements in detection technologies could lead to:

- **Portable detection devices** that doctors can use to monitor the accumulation of graphene in the body in real time.

- **At-home biosensors**, similar to glucose meters, that patients can use independently to monitor their health.

- **Diagnostic imaging technologies** that allow for the non-invasive visualization of nanoparticle accumulation in organs.

Conclusion

The detection of graphene in the human body is a rapidly evolving field. Advanced technologies like Raman spectroscopy, electron microscopy, and mass spectrometry are already providing powerful tools to detect and monitor the presence of graphene nanoparticles in biological tissues. However, access to these technologies is still limited to highly specialized laboratory settings.

With the growing use of graphene across various sectors, including biomedicine, it is essential that research continues to develop more accessible and less invasive monitoring tools. Graphene-based biosensors represent a promising step toward continuous, non-invasive monitoring of nanoparticles in the human body, and in the future, they may become widely available for use in home settings as well.

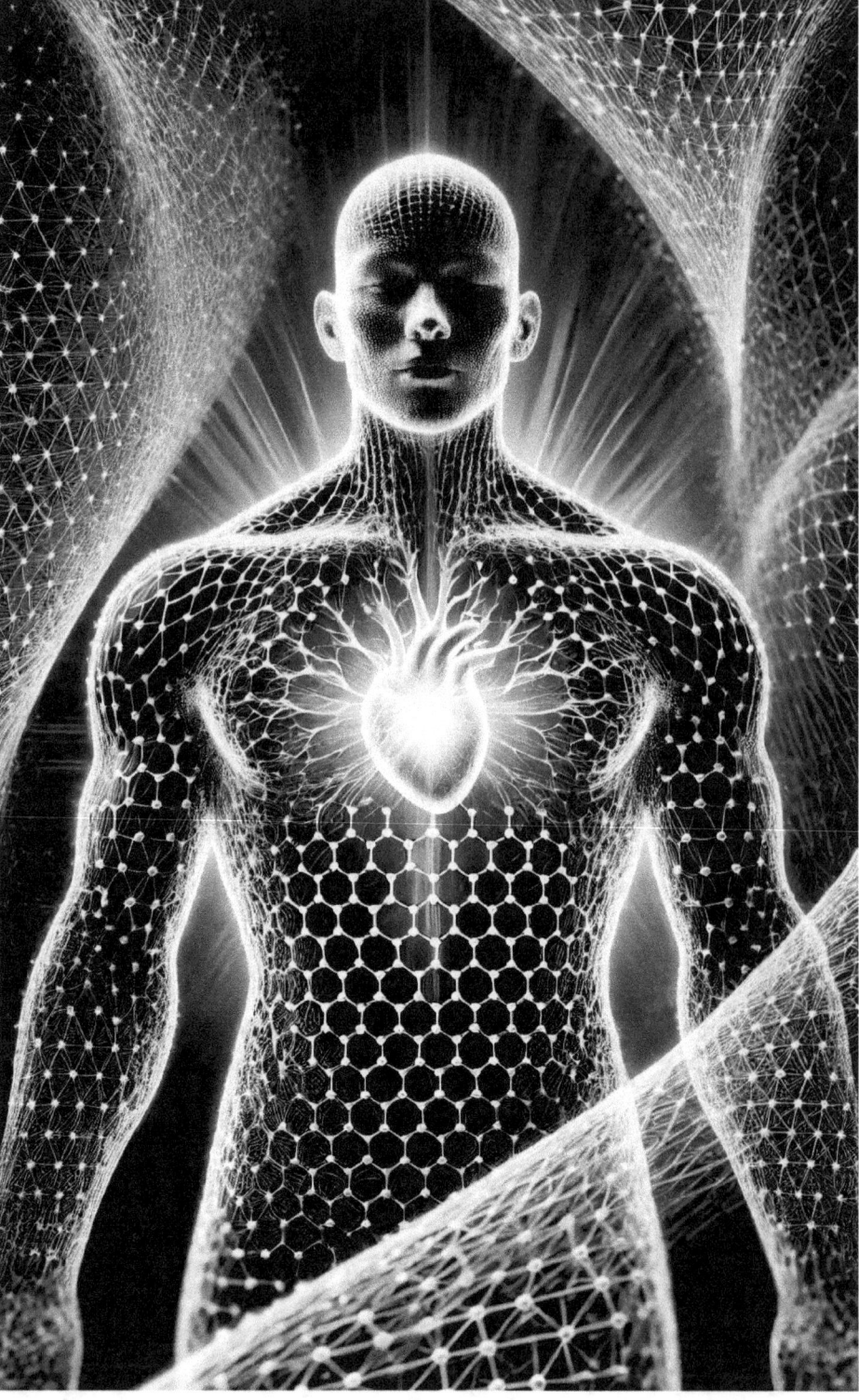

Chapter 4: The Body's Natural Detoxification Mechanisms

The human body has the remarkable ability to naturally eliminate foreign substances through complex biological mechanisms. When it comes to nanoparticles like graphene, the elimination process can be slower and more challenging compared to other substances. However, the immune system, detoxifying organs such as the liver and kidneys, and the lymphatic system all play crucial roles in managing and expelling foreign particles. In this chapter, we will explore the main natural detoxification mechanisms and how the human body can handle graphene nanoparticles.

1. The Immune System: The First Line of Defense

The immune system is the body's first protective barrier against foreign agents, including viruses, bacteria, and nanoparticles like graphene. Immune cells such as macrophages and neutrophils are specialized in recognizing and destroying foreign particles through a process called phagocytosis.

Phagocytosis of Nanoparticles

Phagocytosis is the process by which immune cells engulf and destroy foreign particles. Graphene nanoparticles are recognized by macrophages, which engulf them in an attempt to degrade them. However, because graphene is a highly resilient material, the degradation process can be slow and challenging.

Preclinical studies have shown that graphene oxide particles can accumulate within macrophages, altering their function and leading to chronic inflammation. This can cause tissue damage if the nanoparticle load becomes too high.

A study published in Nature Nanotechnology demonstrated that graphene oxide nanoparticles can become trapped in lung macrophages, preventing them from effectively performing their role. This process can lead to lung inflammation and, in the long term, the formation of scar tissue, known as pulmonary fibrosis.

NK Cells and Graphene

Another key element of the immune system is Natural Killer (NK) cells. These cells are responsible for recognizing and destroying damaged or infected cells. Although NK cells do not directly interact with graphene as macrophages do, they can be activated by the presence of cells damaged by nanoparticles, contributing to the overall immune response.

2. The Liver and Kidneys: The Main Detoxification Organs

The liver and kidneys are two of the most important organs in the detoxification process. They filter the blood, removing toxins and foreign substances, transforming them into compounds that are easier to eliminate.

The Role of the Liver

The liver is the body's primary detoxification organ and plays a crucial role in metabolizing toxic substances. Graphene particles that enter the bloodstream may be transported to the liver, where they are processed through the **cytochrome P450 enzyme system.** This system can break down a wide range of chemical substances, making them water-soluble and easier to excrete. However, unlike many chemical compounds, graphene is structurally resilient and not easily degradable. A study published in Toxicology Letters demonstrated that graphene oxide nanoparticles can accumulate in the liver, causing oxidative damage to liver cells (hepatocytes). The accumulation of high amounts of graphene oxide may induce oxidative stress in the liver, increasing the risk of cellular damage and impairing liver function.

The Role of the Kidneys

The kidneys, on the other hand, are responsible for filtering the blood and excreting toxic substances through urine. Once processed by the liver, graphene is eliminated by the kidneys in the form of metabolites. However, undegraded graphene can accumulate in the kidneys, especially when ingested or inhaled in large quantities.

A study published in Journal of Nanobiotechnology analyzed the renal excretion of graphene oxide nanoparticles in animal models. The results indicated that graphene oxide can become trapped in the renal glomeruli, small structures in the kidneys responsible for blood filtration, potentially leading to long-term kidney damage in cases of prolonged exposure.

3. The Lymphatic System: Toxin Drainage

The lymphatic system is another key player in the process of toxin elimination from the body. It is a network of vessels and lymph nodes that drains body fluids, filters harmful substances, and transports them to the lymph nodes for neutralization. The lymphatic system can play an important role in the transport and removal of graphene nanoparticles from the body.

Lymphatic Drainage and Nanoparticles

Once engulfed by macrophages, graphene nanoparticles can be transported through lymphatic vessels to the lymph nodes, where they are further processed. However, a study published in Biomaterials demonstrated that in some cases, graphene can accumulate in the lymph nodes, causing chronic inflammation and compromising immune function.

The lymphatic system, which drains excess fluids and transports immune cells, is essential for maintaining proper balance in the body. However, when overloaded with nanoparticles, it can become inefficient, delaying the removal of toxins and leading to prolonged inflammation in the tissues.

4. The Elimination of Nanoparticles Through Feces and Urination

Another pathway for eliminating graphene nanoparticles is through the intestines and kidneys, with the excretion of undegraded material via feces and urine.

TIntestinal Excretion

After being processed in the liver, some nanoparticles are excreted into bile and subsequently pass into the intestines, where they are eliminated through feces. This process is particularly important for nanoparticles that cannot be degraded by liver enzymes. A study published in Environmental Science: Nano demonstrated that a significant amount of graphene nanoparticles can be expelled through this route, reducing their accumulation in vital organs.

Urinary Excretion

Urinary excretion is another essential mechanism for eliminating nanoparticles. The kidneys filter the blood and separate unnecessary substances, excreting them through urine. However, due to the small size and structural resilience of graphene, its renal elimination process may be slower compared to other chemical substances.

5. Factors Influencing the Speed of Graphene Elimination

The speed at which graphene is eliminated from the body depends on several factors, including:

- **Particle Size and Shape:** Smaller and irregularly shaped graphene particles tend to accumulate more easily in tissues and are eliminated more slowly.

- **Surface Characteristics:** Nanoparticles functionalized with specific chemical groups may interact more easily with immune system cells and be eliminated more rapidly.

- **Individual Metabolism:** People with faster metabolisms or more efficient liver and kidney function tend to eliminate toxins, including foreign materials like graphene, at a quicker rate.

Conclusion

The human body has sophisticated systems for eliminating foreign substances, including complex materials like graphene. Key organs such as the liver, kidneys, immune system, and lymphatic system work together to expel these nanoparticles, but graphene, due to its size and structural resilience, can pose a particular challenge. Scientific studies have shown that while graphene can be eliminated through pathways such as feces and urine, accumulation in organs like the liver and kidneys may lead to cellular damage and inflammation.

Factors such as the size and shape of the nanoparticles, along with individual liver and kidney function, influence the rate at which graphene is eliminated from the body. However, understanding the natural detoxification mechanisms is the first step toward adopting strategies that can support these processes, minimizing potential health risks.

Further Research and Scientific Studies

- **Nature Nanotechnology – Study on Macrophages and Nanoparticle Accumulation:** This study explores the interaction between graphene oxide nanoparticles and the immune system, showing how graphene can alter macrophage function.

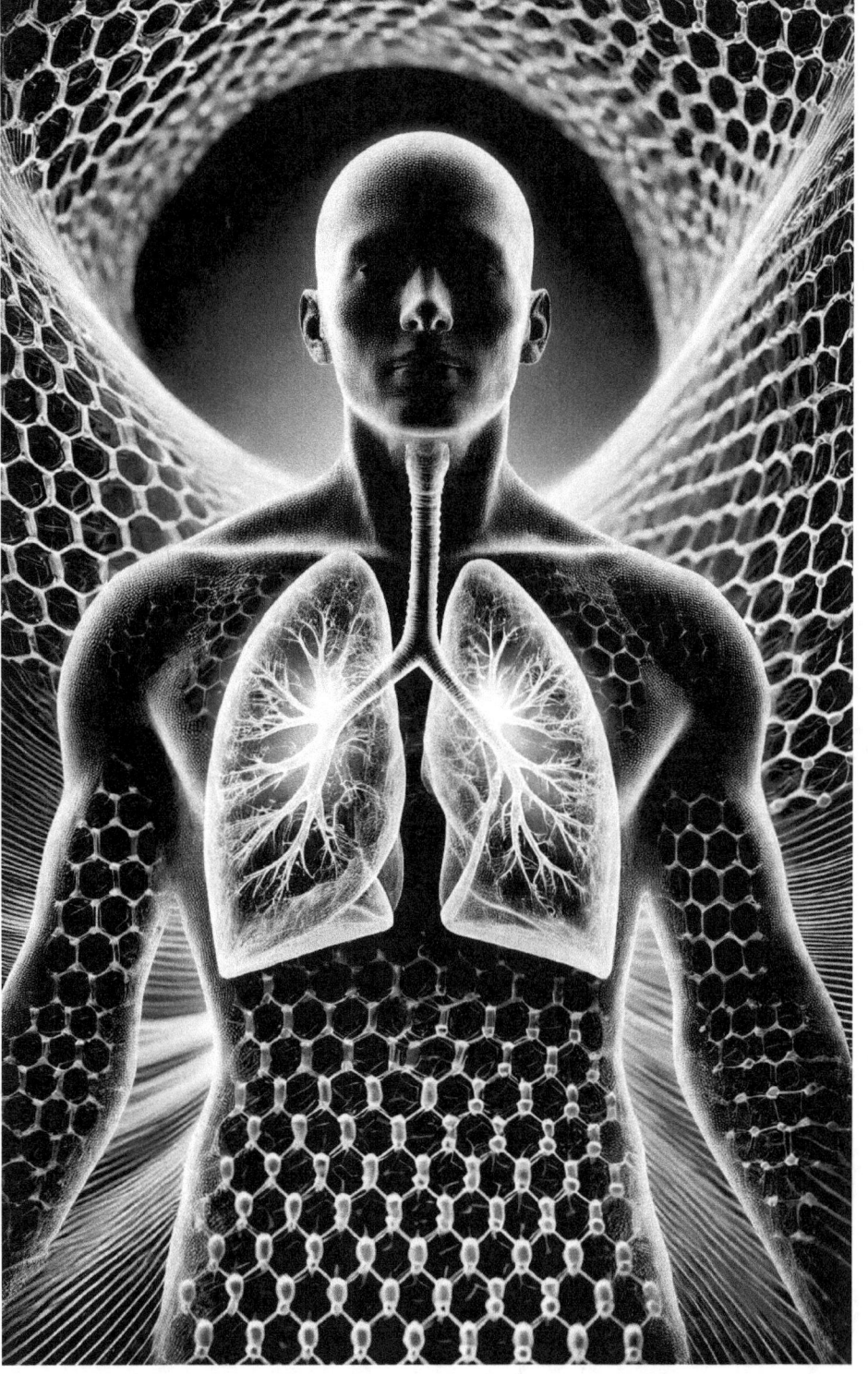

- **Toxicology Letters – Effects of Nanoparticles on the Liver:** This study examined the impact of graphene oxide nanoparticles on the liver, highlighting the risks of oxidative stress and liver damage.

- **Journal of Nanobiotechnology – Study on the Kidneys and Graphene Excretion:** This research explores how graphene can accumulate in the renal glomeruli, leading to potential risks of kidney failure.

- **Environmental Science: Nano – Intestinal Excretion of Graphene:** This study highlights how the body can eliminate graphene through the biliary and intestinal systems.

Chapter 5: Natural Strategies for Detoxifying the Body from Graphene

After exploring the natural mechanisms through which the body eliminates foreign substances like graphene, it's important to understand how to support and optimize this process. Adopting targeted natural strategies can accelerate detoxification and reduce the risk of graphene nanoparticle accumulation in vital organs. In this chapter, we will explore the best natural approaches, including a diet rich in antioxidants, the use of specific supplements, and the adoption of daily practices that promote toxin elimination.

1. Diet as a Detox Tool

One of the simplest and most powerful ways to support the body in the detoxification process is through a targeted diet, rich in nutrients that help neutralize toxins and reduce oxidative stress.

Foods Rich in Antioxidants

Antioxidants are natural compounds that help counteract free radicals and oxidative stress caused by graphene nanoparticles. Including antioxidant-rich foods in your daily diet can improve the body's ability to protect itself from cellular damage.

- **Berries (blueberries, raspberries, blackberries):** These small fruits are known to be rich in antioxidants such as flavonoids, which protect cells from free radical damage. A study published in the Journal of Agricultural and Food Chemistry highlighted that blueberries, in particular, increase antioxidant levels in the body, enhancing liver cell protection and reducing oxidative damage.
- **Leafy green vegetables (spinach, kale):** Leafy greens are rich in vitamins A, C, E, and minerals that help reduce inflammation and improve liver function. Chlorophyll in these vegetables also helps bind toxins and facilitate their elimination.
- **Nuts and seeds:** These foods are rich in vitamin E, which plays an important role in protecting cell membranes from oxidative damage. Regular consumption of nuts (such as Brazil nuts and almonds) can help boost immune system health and reduce the body's toxic load.

Foods with Detoxifying Properties

Some foods have natural detoxifying properties, promoting liver and kidney function.

- **Artichoke:** Known for its liver-protective properties, artichokes contain cynarin, a substance that stimulates bile production and improves liver function. Studies conducted on patients with liver issues have shown that artichoke extract helps regenerate the liver and enhance toxin elimination.

- **Dandelion:** Dandelion is one of the most commonly used herbs for liver and kidney detoxification. It stimulates bile production and promotes toxin elimination through urine. Regular use of dandelion tea can help support the detoxification process, as indicated by a study published in the Journal of Ethnopharmacology.

Sample Detox Diet Plan

Here is an example of a weekly diet plan that can be adopted to improve graphene detoxification and reduce oxidative stress:

- **Breakfast:** Blueberry, spinach, chia seed, and almond milk smoothie. This mix provides antioxidants, fiber, and healthy fats.
- **Lunch:** Kale salad with avocado, pumpkin seeds, and extra virgin olive oil. Add steamed artichokes for enhanced detoxifying properties.
- **Dinner:** Grilled salmon with broccoli and quinoa. Salmon provides Omega-3s to reduce inflammation, while broccoli contains compounds that stimulate the liver.
- **Snacks**: Brazil nuts (rich in selenium) and dandelion tea.

2. Essential Supplements for Detoxifying the Body from Graphene

In addition to diet, certain natural supplements can support liver and kidney function, enhancing the body's ability to eliminate graphene nanoparticles.

Glutathione

Glutathione is one of the most powerful antioxidants in the body, and it plays a particularly important role in the liver, the main organ responsible for detoxification. Glutathione helps neutralize toxins and facilitates their elimination from the body.

A study published in Free Radical Biology & Medicine demonstrated that taking glutathione supplements can increase the body's capacity to detoxify graphene nanoparticles, improving liver function and reducing oxidative damage.

N-acetylcysteine (NAC)

N-acetylcysteine (NAC) is a precursor to glutathione and has been shown to be effective in supporting the body's production of this important antioxidant. NAC is frequently used to support liver detoxification and reduce inflammation.

A study conducted on animals and published in Toxicology and Applied Pharmacology found that NAC helps protect liver cells from damage induced by graphene nanoparticles, improving their elimination through the kidneys.

Milk Thistle

Milk thistle is an herb known for its liver-protective properties, thanks to its active component, **silymarin**. This substance helps protect liver cells from toxic damage and promotes liver regeneration. A study published in Journal of Hepatology demonstrated that milk thistle can reduce the accumulation of toxic substances in the liver, facilitating their elimination.

Zeolite

Zeolite is a natural mineral that can bind to toxins, including heavy metals and nanoparticles, promoting their excretion. Many proponents of natural detoxification use zeolite to support the removal of particles like graphene from the body. Although specific studies on graphene are lacking, zeolite's ability to bind to other nanoparticles makes it a promising candidate.

3. The Importance of Hydration and Physical Activity

Water and physical activity are two key elements in supporting the body's detoxification process.

Effective Hydration

Drinking sufficient amounts of water is essential to help the kidneys filter out toxins. A consistent intake of water ensures that harmful substances are eliminated through urine. It is important to drink at least 8 glasses of water per day, increasing intake during periods of higher exposure to toxins or while following detoxification plans.

Water also helps maintain fluid balance in the body, facilitates digestion, and supports the lymphatic system, which is crucial for draining toxins.

Regular Physical Exercise

Physical activity increases blood flow and stimulates metabolism, accelerating the detoxification process. Exercises such as light jogging, swimming, and cycling can help the body expel toxins through sweat, improving overall health.

A regular exercise routine also helps reduce stress levels, an important factor since chronic stress can slow down detoxification processes.

4. Detoxifying Teas and Drinks

Detoxifying teas are a powerful and natural tool for supporting liver and kidney function and promoting toxin elimination. In addition to dandelion and milk thistle teas, many other beverages offer similar benefits. Green tea, rich in antioxidants, is particularly effective in helping the body combat oxidative stress caused by nanoparticles such as graphene.

Green Tea

Green tea is well-known for its high antioxidant content, especially polyphenols and catechins, which protect cells from oxidative damage and stimulate metabolism. A study published in The Journal of Nutrition highlighted that green tea catechins increase the antioxidant capacity of the blood and improve liver detoxification. Green tea also helps protect the liver from chemical toxin-induced damage and may facilitate liver cell regeneration.

Ginger Tea

Ginger is a root with anti-inflammatory and antioxidant properties that can support digestion and promote detoxification. It stimulates blood circulation and bile flow, thus aiding in the elimination of toxins through the liver. A study published in Food & Function showed that ginger has protective effects on the liver and can help reduce oxidative stress levels.

Turmeric Tea

Turmeric is a spice with potent antioxidant properties, thanks to its active component, curcumin. Curcumin is known for its anti-inflammatory effects and its support of liver detoxification. A study published in Liver International demonstrated that curcumin may help prevent liver damage induced by toxic substances, improving the body's ability to safely eliminate them.

Fennel Tea

Fennel is a plant with diuretic properties that helps improve kidney function and eliminate toxins through urine. Additionally, fennel can stimulate digestion and reduce abdominal bloating, enhancing the efficiency of the digestive system and supporting the removal of toxic substances. Fennel tea is particularly useful for those looking to support kidney function during a detox process.

Lemon Water

Lemon water is another excellent tool for stimulating detoxification. Lemon juice, rich in vitamin C and antioxidants, helps cleanse the liver and stimulates bile production, which is essential for toxin elimination. Drinking warm lemon water in the morning can improve digestion and prepare the body for an effective day of detoxification.

5. Breathing Techniques and Saunas for Toxin Elimination

In addition to diet and supplements, there are natural techniques that can enhance toxin elimination. Deep breathing techniques, saunas, and steam baths are effective tools for stimulating metabolism and eliminating toxins through sweat and respiration.

Deep Breathing

Deep breathing stimulates the lymphatic system and improves the body's oxygenation. This process can help the body eliminate toxins through exhalation and reduce oxidative stress. Practicing deep breathing techniques daily, such as pranayama or diaphragmatic breathing, can enhance lymphatic function and improve blood circulation.

Saunas and Steam Baths

Saunas and steam baths are effective methods for stimulating sweating, one of the primary ways the body eliminates toxins. Sweating helps cleanse the skin and remove accumulated harmful chemicals, including nanoparticles. A study published in the Journal of Environmental and Public Health showed that sweating induced by regular sauna use can facilitate the elimination of heavy metals and other toxins from the body.

The use of **infrared saunas**, in particular, has been suggested as a method to eliminate toxins at the cellular level, as the heat penetrates more deeply into the tissues compared to traditional saunas.

6. Detoxification and Reducing Oxidative Stress

Reducing oxidative stress is crucial in the detoxification process, as prolonged stress can compromise the immune system and slow the body's ability to eliminate toxins like graphene. In addition to diet and supplements, there are practices that can reduce oxidative stress and improve overall health.

Rest and Sleep Quality

Quality sleep is essential for allowing the body to regenerate and repair itself during the night. During sleep, the body carries out many of its detoxification and cellular repair functions. A lack of sleep can slow down the toxin elimination process and increase inflammation levels.

Ensuring you get 7-8 hours of sleep per night and establishing a relaxing evening routine with good sleep hygiene can significantly improve natural detoxification.

Stress Reduction

Chronic stress can negatively affect the detoxification process by increasing cortisol levels, the stress hormone, which can impair liver function. Daily practice of stress management techniques such as meditation, yoga, and progressive muscle relaxation can reduce oxidative stress and improve the body's ability to eliminate toxins.

Conclusion

In this chapter, we have explored various natural strategies to support the body in the detoxification process from graphene. Through a combination of diet, supplements, hydration, physical exercise, and relaxation practices, it is possible to help the body reduce oxidative stress and improve the efficiency of nanoparticle elimination. Adopting these strategies not only helps protect the body from the potential consequences of graphene accumulation but also promotes overall well-being, enhancing long-term health.

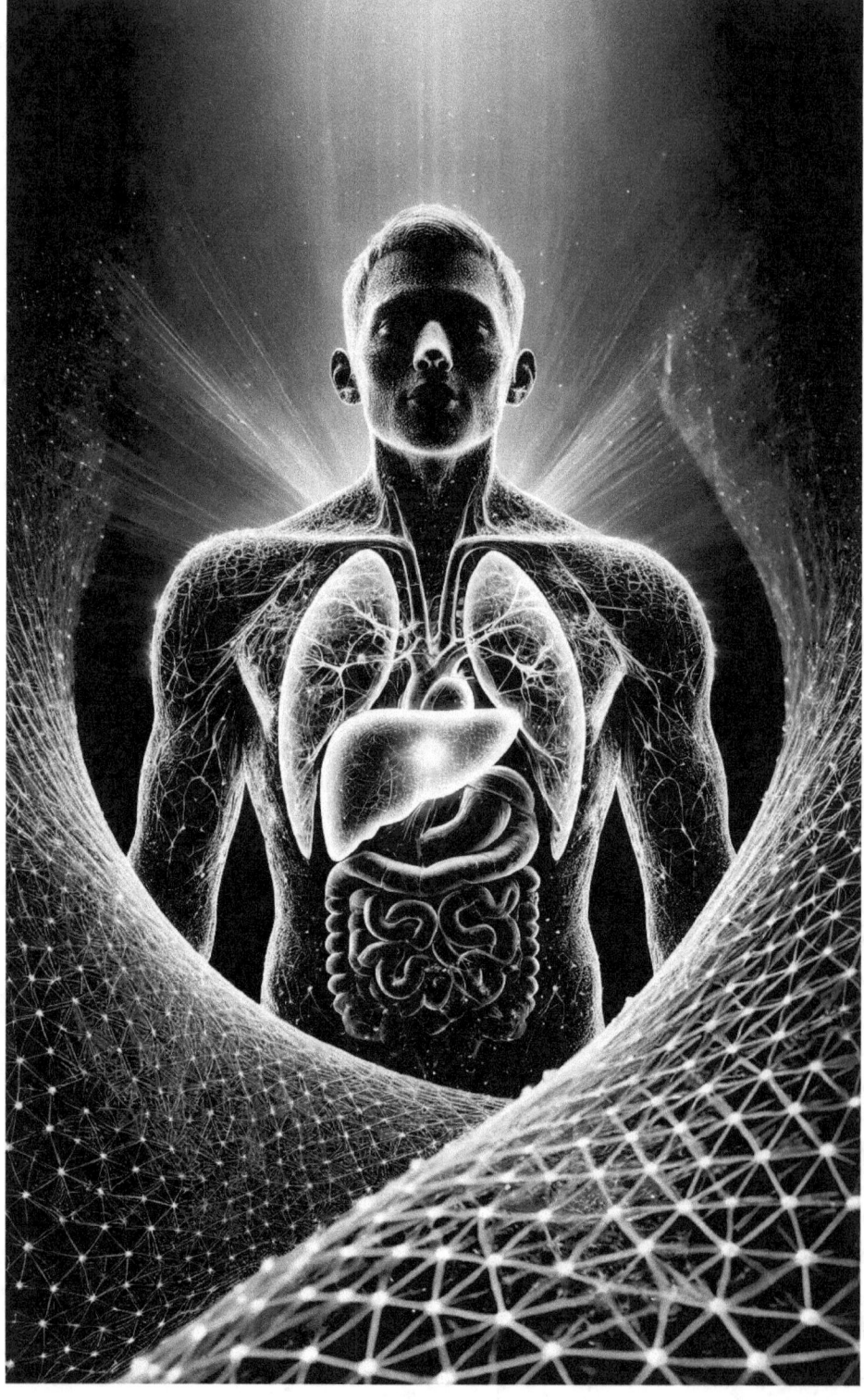

Chapter 6: Success Stories and Testimonials

The natural detoxification strategies described in the previous chapters are supported not only by science but also by real-life testimonials from people who have followed effective detoxification plans and experienced improvements in their health. This chapter gathers success stories from individuals who have adopted detoxification practices and integrated natural approaches into their daily lives to address exposure to substances like graphene. These experiences, based on case studies and testimonials, demonstrate how a holistic approach can enhance overall well-being and facilitate the elimination of toxins.

1. Case Study: Peter E. - Improvement in Liver and Kidney Function

Peter, a 42-year-old man, began experiencing chronic fatigue and persistent digestive problems after environmental exposure to toxic substances while working in an industrial sector. After learning about the potential toxicity of nanoparticles like graphene, he decided to pursue a natural detoxification plan to improve his health.

Detoxification Strategy

Peter followed a diet rich in antioxidants and supplemented with glutathione and N-acetylcysteine (NAC) to enhance liver function. He included foods such as blueberries, spinach, and nuts in his diet and started drinking dandelion and milk thistle teas daily to support liver functionality.

After just three months, Peter noticed a significant improvement in his energy levels, a reduction in abdominal bloating, and improved kidney function. His blood tests showed a reduction in markers of liver inflammation, suggesting that his detoxification plan was effectively helping to remove toxins from his body.

2. Case Study: Clare G. - Toxin Removal and Respiratory Health Improvement

Clare, a 55-year-old woman, experienced prolonged exposure to graphene nanoparticles through the inhalation of fine dust in an industrial setting. After she began experiencing respiratory issues, including shortness of breath and frequent fatigue, she turned to a natural approach to improve her lung health.

Clare Approach

Clare incorporated anti-inflammatory and detoxifying foods into her diet, such as ginger and turmeric. She also began practicing deep breathing exercises regularly and used an infrared sauna to stimulate sweating and the elimination of toxins through her skin.

After six months, Clare experienced a significant reduction in her respiratory symptoms and reported an improvement in lung capacity, as confirmed by medical tests. Her story demonstrates that detoxification techniques, including dietary interventions and relaxation and purification methods, can improve lung health.

3. Case Study: Mark T. - Improvement in Mental Clarity

Mark, 38, suffered from "brain fog," a condition characterized by difficulty concentrating and mental fatigue, which developed after exposure to graphene nanoparticles in a technological research setting. Feeling limited in his cognitive abilities, he began a specific detoxification program to improve neurological function.

Mark Journey

Mark adopted a diet rich in Omega-3 fatty acids, found in foods like salmon and flaxseeds, and supplemented his diet with glutathione to reduce brain inflammation. He also began practicing yoga and meditation to manage stress and support neuronal detoxification.

After three months, Mark reported a significant improvement in his ability to concentrate and mental clarity. His experience highlights the importance of incorporating dietary interventions and mindful lifestyle practices to support neurological function during a detoxification process.

4. Testimonial: Adele M. - Reduction in Fatigue Symptoms and Renewed Energy

Adele, 45, had been suffering from chronic fatigue and irritability for several months, attributing her symptoms to toxin buildup and exposure to industrial chemicals. After consulting with natural health experts, she decided to follow a detoxification plan that included natural supplements and a diet rich in antioxidants.

Adele Detox Plan

Adele began taking NAC supplements and adopted a diet rich in berries, leafy green vegetables, and seeds. She also incorporated detoxifying drinks into her daily routine, such as green tea and turmeric infusions, to reduce inflammation.

After several months, Adele noticed a marked improvement in her daily energy levels, feeling less fatigued and more active. Her lab results showed reduced inflammation and improved liver function. Her story highlights the effectiveness of an antioxidant-rich diet combined with natural supplements to enhance overall well-being.

5. Testimonial: Denis W. - The Role of Sauna and Hydration in Detoxification

Denis, 50, experienced accidental exposure to graphene nanoparticles in a laboratory and began suffering from recurring headaches and muscle aches. He turned to detoxification practices that included the use of infrared saunas and a strict hydration routine.

Denis Detoxification Journey

Denis started using an infrared sauna three times a week, combining the sessions with a hydration regime that included electrolyte-rich water and detoxifying teas such as fennel and dandelion tea. After six months, Denis reported a significant reduction in his physical symptoms, including improved muscle aches and the disappearance of his headaches. He also noticed increased vitality and mental clarity. His testimonial highlights the importance of using saunas and effective hydration to promote the elimination of accumulated toxins in the body.

Conclusion

The success stories presented in this chapter demonstrate how a natural and holistic approach can improve overall health and facilitate the elimination of toxins, including graphene nanoparticles. Through a combination of diet, supplements, hydration, and purification techniques like saunas and deep breathing, many individuals have achieved tangible improvements in their health. Their detoxification journeys offer valuable insights for those seeking natural solutions to protect their bodies from toxic substances and enhance long-term well-being. In the coming chapters, we will explore emerging research and new technologies for detecting and managing nanoparticles in the human body.

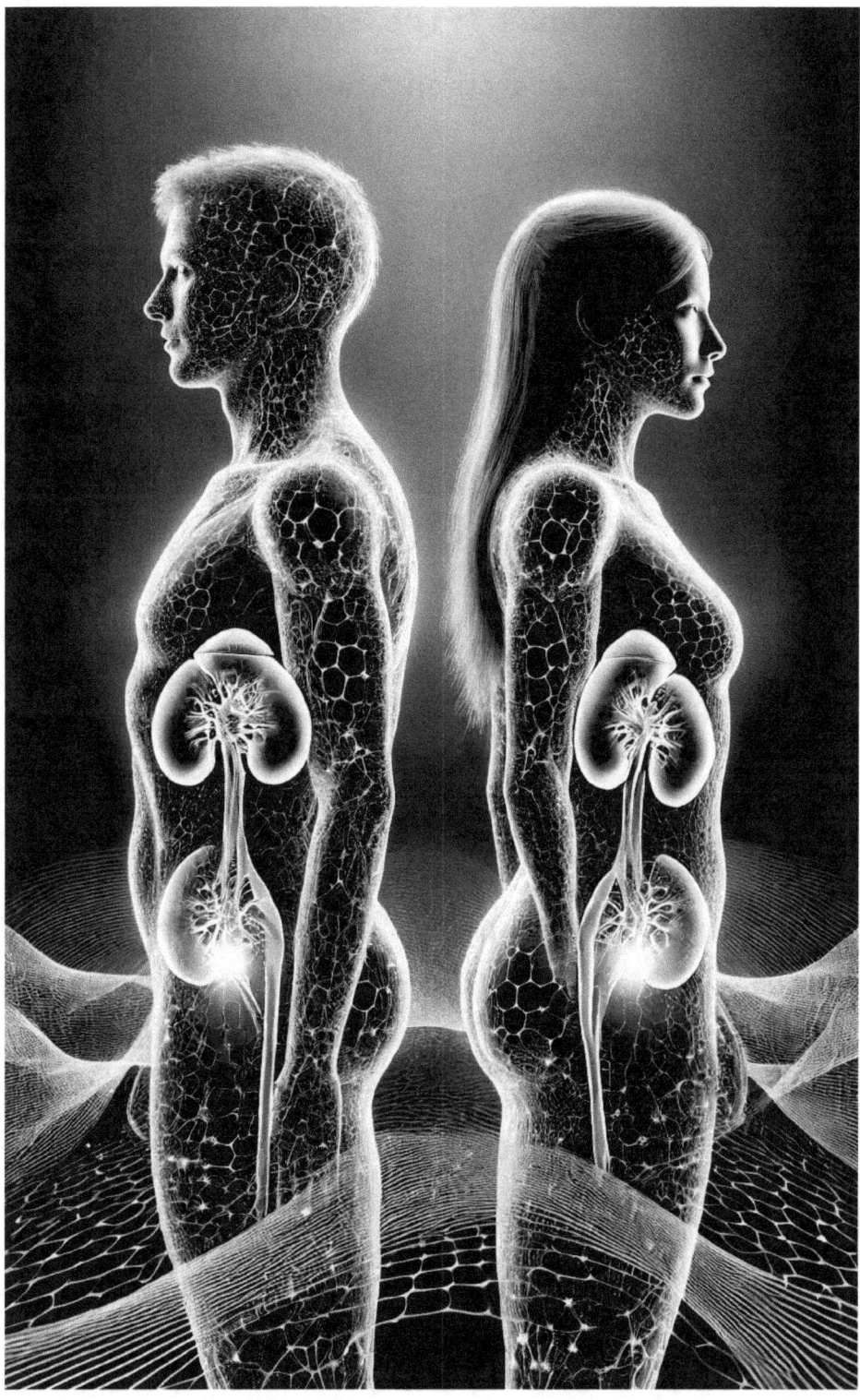

Chapter 7: The Evolving Research on Graphene

The science of graphene is constantly evolving, with new discoveries emerging each year regarding its properties and its impact on human health. While graphene is praised for its technological potential, research is increasingly focusing on its biological effects, particularly to better understand the risks associated with exposure and to develop new methods for its safe elimination from the body. In this chapter, we will explore the latest scientific studies and advancements in understanding the interaction between graphene and the human body, as well as emerging innovations in the field of nanomedicine.

1. The Biological Effects of Graphene: New Discoveries

The effects of graphene on the human body are a topic of growing interest in the scientific community. Recent research has made significant progress in understanding how graphene nanoparticles interact with cells and tissues, shedding light on the potential toxic effects and the mechanisms by which the body attempts to manage their elimination.

Molecular and Cellular Level Effects

A study published in Small explored the molecular effects of graphene oxide (GO) nanoparticles on cellular membranes. Researchers discovered that GO can destabilize cell membranes, causing structural integrity loss and leading to cell death through necrosis or apoptosis. These effects were especially observed in lung and liver cells, raising concerns about prolonged inhalation and the accumulation of graphene in tissues.

Additionally, a study in Toxicology Research suggested that graphene can induce an inflammatory response in immune system cells. Macrophages, responsible for phagocytosing foreign substances, appear unable to fully degrade graphene, which can lead to chronic inflammation in tissues where these nanoparticles accumulate. This finding raises questions about the long-term use of graphene in industrial and technological environments and the possible consequences for workers exposed to it.

Influence of Graphene's Chemical Surface

A crucial aspect of graphene studies is how modifications to its chemical surface affect its biocompatibility.

Particles functionalized with specific chemical groups seem to interact differently with cells compared to non-functionalized particles. A study in *Nature Communications* demonstrated that surface functionalization of graphene can reduce its toxicity, making it safer for use in medical applications. This opens the door to the development of new, less harmful versions of graphene for the human body.

2. Nanomedicine: Graphene as a Therapeutic Tool

While much of the research focuses on the potential harmful effects of graphene, another avenue is exploring how this material can be used for therapeutic purposes. Nanomedicine, which utilizes nanoparticles to deliver drugs or monitor biological parameters, is an emerging field investigating the use of graphene in various medical contexts.

Graphene as a Drug Carrier

One of the most promising areas of research is the use of graphene as a carrier for controlled drug release. Due to its large surface area and ability to be functionalized with bioactive molecules, graphene could be used to deliver drugs directly to diseased cells, reducing side effects and increasing therapeutic efficacy.

A study published in Biomaterials showed that graphene oxide functionalized with anticancer molecules can transport chemotherapy drugs directly into cancer cells, improving the treatment's effectiveness.

Graphene in Diagnostic Devices

Another area of interest is the development of graphene-based biosensors for real-time patient health monitoring. Since graphene is extremely sensitive to electrical and chemical variations, it is an ideal material for creating sensors that can detect changes in blood biomarkers or body fluids. Recent studies have developed graphene sensors capable of monitoring glucose levels in diabetic patients or detecting the presence of viruses and bacteria quickly and efficiently.

These advancements in nanomedicine suggest that, while graphene poses a potential risk when inhaled or ingested in large quantities, its controlled use in therapeutic applications could offer enormous health benefits.

3. Emerging Research on the Mechanisms of Graphene Elimination

One of the main current challenges is understanding how the body can effectively eliminate graphene once it accumulates in tissues. While the human body has powerful detoxification mechanisms, graphene presents a unique challenge due to its resilience and nanometric size.

The Role of the Immune System in Graphene Elimination

A recent study in the Journal of Nanobiotechnology highlighted how the immune system reacts to the presence of graphene nanoparticles. Macrophages, the cells responsible for engulfing and degrading foreign substances, can phagocytose graphene, but complete degradation is ineffective. The accumulation of these particles within macrophages can lead to chronic inflammatory responses, particularly in the lungs and liver.

Another study examined how surface functionalization of graphene could improve the body's ability to eliminate it through the lymphatic and renal systems. This line of research suggests that chemically modifying graphene may facilitate its expulsion through urine or the lymphatic system, reducing tissue accumulation and minimizing long-term damage.

Future Therapies to Facilitate Graphene Elimination

An exciting area of research involves developing specific molecules or enzymes capable of binding to graphene and facilitating its elimination. Some studies are investigating the use of bioactive nanoparticles that can "cut" graphene nanoparticles into smaller fragments, which can be more easily expelled from the body through the kidneys.

4. Future Innovations in Graphene Research

The future of graphene research is promising and multidisciplinary, with increasing interest from fields such as medicine, technology, and energy. Collaborations between material scientists, biologists, doctors, and engineers are accelerating the development of innovative technologies that can harness the unique properties of graphene for safe and effective medical applications.

Graphene and Advanced Biocompatibility

One line of research is exploring how to further improve the biocompatibility of graphene. The goal is to develop modified versions of graphene that can be used in medical implants or biosensors without triggering an inflammatory response or accumulating in tissues. Studies on functionalized nanoparticles suggest that, in the future, graphene could be used in a wide range of medical applications, from monitoring devices for chronic patients to targeted cancer treatments.

Conclusion

Graphene research is continuously evolving, with new discoveries shedding light on both the risks and benefits of its use in the biomedical field. While it is clear that uncontrolled exposure to graphene can pose health risks, emerging research is paving the way for new solutions to manage these risks and harness graphene's therapeutic potential safely.

Innovations in nanomedicine and research on the mechanisms of graphene elimination offer new hopes for the future, suggesting that graphene could become a valuable ally in modern medicine, provided it is handled responsibly and supported by scientific evidence.

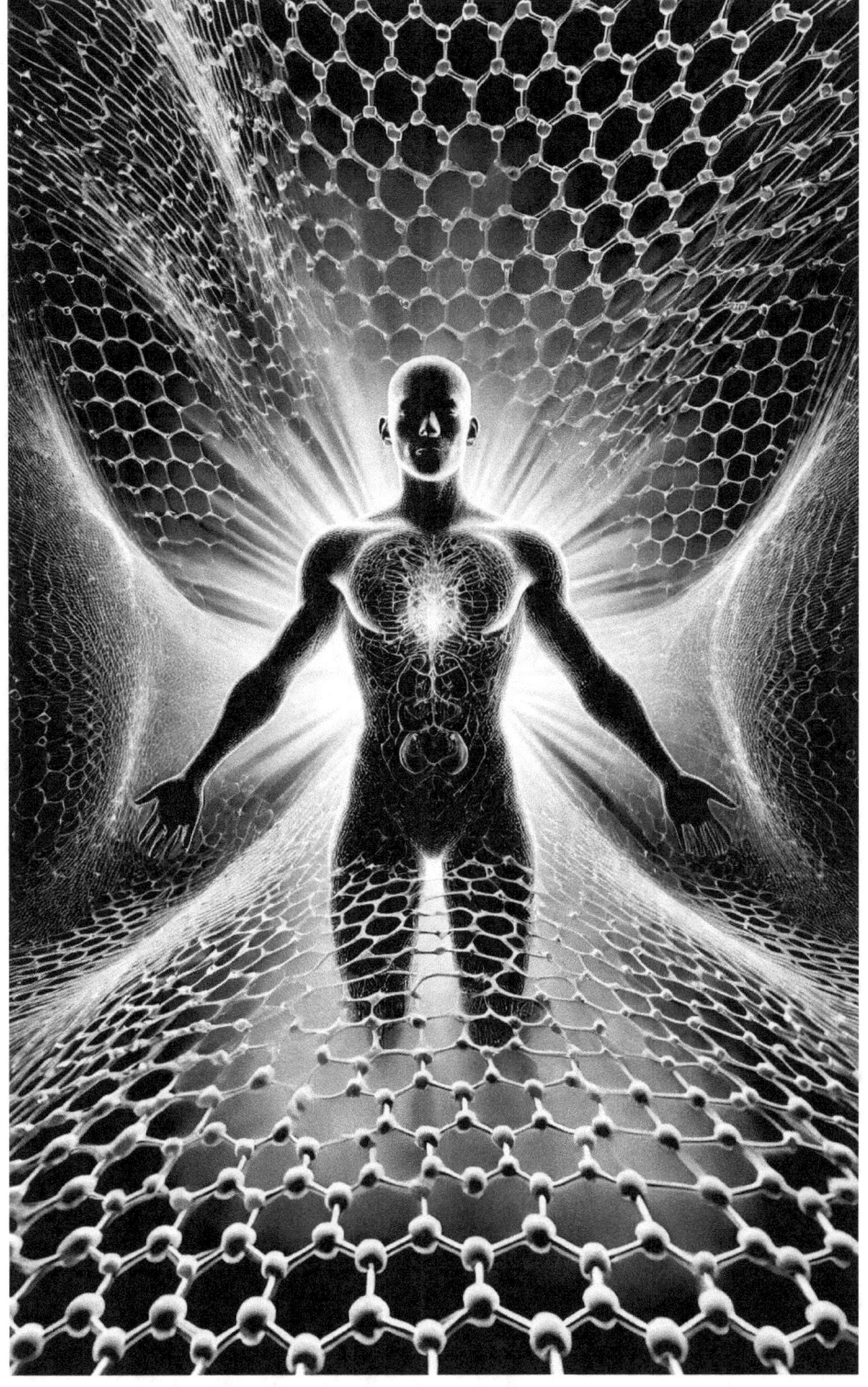

Chapter 8: Tools for Health Monitoring and Home Evaluation

Monitoring one's health is essential to understanding how the body reacts to toxin accumulation, including materials like graphene. Fortunately, modern technology has made advanced tools available that allow individuals to monitor their exposure to nanoparticles and assess their health status directly from home. In this chapter, we will explore the various devices, techniques, and practices that can help identify potential issues related to toxin buildup and improve overall well-being.

1. Health Monitoring through Wearable Devices

Wearable devices are technological tools that allow continuous monitoring of vital signs such as heart rate, blood oxygen levels, and other health indicators. These devices provide an opportunity to detect any physiological anomalies that could be related to the accumulation of toxins or nanoparticles in the body, including graphene.

Wearable Devices and Toxin Detection

An emerging field of research focuses on the development of wearable biosensors that can monitor toxin levels in the blood and bodily fluids.

These devices can detect changes in biochemical parameters that indicate the presence of foreign materials, such as graphene nanoparticles, or markers of oxidative stress caused by the accumulation of such materials.

A study published in Nano Letters demonstrated the effectiveness of graphene-based biosensors for real-time health monitoring. Due to its high sensitivity, graphene is used to develop sensors capable of detecting even the smallest changes in biomarkers, thus enabling the monitoring of exposure to toxic substances and the body's inflammatory responses.

Commercial Wearable Devices

Some of the most common wearable devices, like fitness trackers (e.g., Fitbit or Apple Watch), monitor heart rate, sleep quality, and blood oxygen levels. These parameters can be useful in detecting imbalances or signs of physical or mental fatigue, which may be associated with the buildup of toxins or nanoparticles. While not specifically designed to detect graphene, these tools provide a general overview of health that can help identify issues related to prolonged exposure to toxic substances.

2. Self-Assessment Tests and Home Monitoring

In addition to wearable devices, there are tests and tools that can be used at home to monitor the presence of toxins and nanoparticles in the body. These self-assessment tools can provide valuable data to assess the accumulation of graphene or other chemicals.

Glutathione and Antioxidant Level Testing

Since glutathione is one of the main antioxidants responsible for the body's detoxification, measuring glutathione levels in the blood or urine can be an effective way to evaluate the body's ability to eliminate toxins like graphene. Some home tests, such as urine analysis kits for glutathione, are commercially available and can provide insight into the body's natural detoxification status.

A study in Free Radical Research highlighted that lower levels of glutathione are often correlated with increased oxidative damage and a reduced ability to eliminate toxins. Regularly monitoring these levels can help determine if the body is successfully managing the accumulation of graphene nanoparticles and other toxic materials.

Immune System Monitoring Tests

Another important health indicator is the immune system. Tests to monitor inflammation levels in the body, such as measuring C-reactive protein (CRP), can be performed at home using blood test kits. Elevated CRP levels indicate a state of chronic inflammation, which could be related to the accumulation of graphene nanoparticles in tissues.

Heavy Metal and Nanoparticle Monitoring Tests

Some home monitoring kits allow for the detection of heavy metals in the body, such as mercury or lead, which are often correlated with nanoparticle accumulation. While specific tests to detect graphene at home are not yet available, these tests can provide a general overview of toxic substance accumulation in the body and indicate a need for detoxification.

3. Home Toxin Detection Techniques

There are also indirect detection techniques that can be used at home to assess potential toxin accumulation in the body. While these techniques may not be as precise as laboratory tests, they can provide useful indicators for monitoring overall health.

Skin and Mucous Membrane Check-ups

The body often signals toxin accumulation through the skin. Regularly examining the skin for signs of irritation, redness, or rashes can be a way to monitor health. A study in the Journal of Dermatological Science highlighted that the buildup of heavy metals and other nanoparticles can cause inflammation and dermatological disorders. These signs may indicate overexposure to substances like graphene and necessitate detoxification interventions.

Monitoring Respiratory Function

Since graphene can accumulate in the lungs if inhaled, regularly monitoring lung capacity can provide valuable information about respiratory health. Home devices such as portable spirometers can be used to measure lung function and detect any decreases in respiratory capacity, which could indicate inflammation or lung damage caused by nanoparticle buildup.

A study published in the American Journal of Respiratory and Critical Care Medicine demonstrated that exposure to nanoparticles can reduce lung function, and regular monitoring can help identify problems early.

4. The Importance of Regular Medical Evaluations

While home tests and wearable devices can provide useful information, it is essential to supplement them with regular medical evaluations. Healthcare professionals can perform more in-depth and precise tests, such as Raman spectroscopy or electron microscopy, to detect the presence of graphene nanoparticles in tissues. These examinations are crucial for confirming any hypotheses based on data collected at home.

Advanced Imaging Examinations

In addition to lab tests, advanced imaging techniques such as computed tomography (CT) and magnetic resonance imaging (MRI) can detect inflammation and abnormalities in the lungs or liver caused by nanoparticle accumulation. These exams, combined with biochemical tests, provide a comprehensive health assessment and help determine the need for more specific detoxification interventions.

5. Final Recommendations for Home Health Monitoring (continued)

To best manage your health and prevent the accumulation of toxins like graphene, the following additional steps are recommended:

4. Adopt a Healthy Lifestyle

Supporting natural detoxification processes through a diet rich in antioxidants, regular physical activity, and relaxation techniques is essential. Consuming foods high in vitamin C, E, and glutathione (such as fruits and vegetables) helps reduce oxidative stress and boosts the immune system, facilitating the elimination of toxins like graphene. Exercise improves blood circulation and metabolism, speeding up the process of removing nanoparticles through sweat and urine. Practices like yoga and meditation can also help reduce stress, promoting overall mental and physical well-being.

5. Increase Hydration and Consume Detoxifying Beverages

Drinking plenty of water is crucial to keeping the kidneys active and supporting the body's detoxification process. As discussed in previous chapters, detoxifying teas such as dandelion, milk thistle, or green tea can help stimulate the liver and kidneys, facilitating the elimination of toxic substances like graphene nanoparticles. These beverages support the body in reducing inflammation and promoting cellular regeneration.

6. Supplement with Specific Detoxification Nutrients

Natural supplements such as glutathione, N-acetylcysteine (NAC), milk thistle, and zeolite can be used to enhance the body's ability to eliminate toxins. These supplements support liver and kidney function, reducing the toxic load on the body and promoting the regeneration of damaged cells.

7. Monitor Symptoms and Signs of Toxin Accumulation

It is important to pay attention to warning signs from the body, such as chronic fatigue, digestive issues, brain fog, respiratory problems, skin rashes, or inflammation. These symptoms may indicate a toxic overload, such as from graphene, and may require more aggressive detoxification measures or prompt medical consultation.

8. Maintain Good Environmental Hygiene

Reducing exposure to graphene nanoparticles or other toxic substances can start with the home environment. Using air purifiers to remove airborne particles and regularly cleaning surfaces can reduce the buildup of toxins in the home. Additionally, avoiding the use of industrial or household products containing nanoparticles helps reduce accidental exposure.

9. Consult Health Professionals for Specialized Monitoring

If there are suspicions of prolonged exposure or graphene accumulation, it is advisable to consult a doctor or a toxicology expert. Some doctors may recommend more advanced tests, such as mass spectrometry or Raman spectroscopy, to assess the presence of nanoparticles in the body and provide specific guidance on treatment and detoxification.

Conclusion

In this chapter, we explored various tools and techniques for home health monitoring and the prevention of toxic nanoparticle accumulation, such as graphene. Using wearable devices, self-assessment tests, and monitoring tools, combined with a healthy lifestyle and regular medical consultations, can provide a clear overview of your health status and the body's ability to manage toxins. Adopting these practices not only improves daily well-being but also helps prevent problems related to prolonged nanoparticle exposure, ensuring long-term protection for the body.

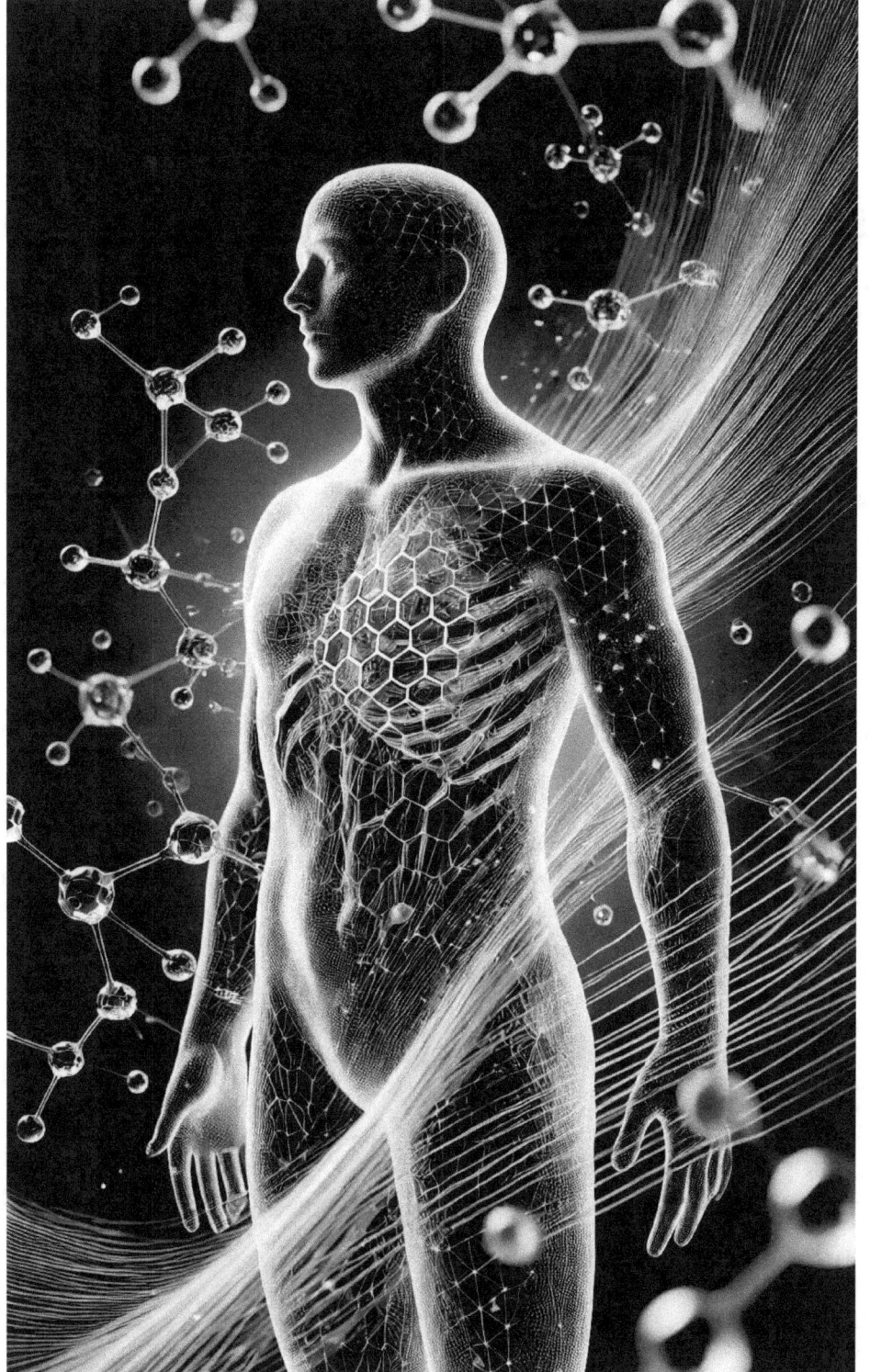

Chapter 9: Future Innovations and Potential Drugs for Graphene

In recent years, science has made significant strides in understanding the effects of graphene on the human body. At the same time, new technologies and therapies are being developed to help the body manage the accumulation of nanoparticles like graphene. This chapter focuses on emerging innovations in scientific and medical research that could offer new solutions for managing nanoparticles in the body, with a particular emphasis on cutting-edge drugs and technologies for detoxification.

1. Potential Drugs for Neutralizing Graphene

One of the most innovative approaches to managing graphene in the body involves the development of specialized drugs capable of binding to graphene nanoparticles, reducing their toxic effects, and facilitating their elimination.

Bioactive Molecules and Enhanced Antioxidants

Many studies are exploring the use of bioactive molecules and advanced antioxidants to reduce oxidative stress induced by graphene and neutralize its harmful effects.

A promising candidate is superoxide dismutase (SOD), an enzyme that acts as an antioxidant and could be administered in drug form to combat the accumulation of reactive oxygen species (ROS) caused by graphene nanoparticles. A study published in Free Radical Biology & Medicine demonstrated that increasing SOD levels in the body can significantly reduce cellular damage caused by graphene nanoparticles, promoting cellular regeneration. Integrating this bioactive molecule could be a key therapeutic strategy to mitigate the negative effects of graphene in tissues.

Drugs that Promote Renal Excretion

Another promising area of research focuses on the development of drugs that enhance kidney function and stimulate the excretion of graphene nanoparticles through urine. Researchers are working on molecules capable of binding to the nanoparticles and making them more soluble, thereby facilitating their transport through the kidneys and their elimination. A study published in the Journal of Nanomedicine showed that specific drugs can be used to increase the solubility of graphene oxide nanoparticles, reducing the risk of renal accumulation and improving urinary excretion. These drugs could represent a practical solution to prevent kidney damage and reduce the toxic load in the body.

2. Nanotechnologies for the Removal of Nanoparticles

Beyond pharmaceuticals, the field of nanotechnology offers new possibilities for treating and eliminating graphene in the body. These innovations focus on miniaturized tools and technologies capable of more efficiently monitoring and neutralizing nanoparticles.

Enzymatic Nanoparticles

One of the most promising innovations involves the development of enzymatic nanoparticles capable of degrading graphene nanoparticles in the body. These specialized nanoparticles are designed to bind to graphene and break it down into smaller fragments that can be easily eliminated. These synthetic enzymes are designed to be biocompatible and act without damaging surrounding cells.

A study published in Nature Nanotechnology demonstrated that enzymatic nanoparticles can significantly reduce the graphene load in the body, decreasing inflammation and facilitating the regeneration of damaged tissues. This approach could represent a breakthrough in the management of nanoparticles in medical settings, offering a safe and effective method for detoxification.

Nanocapsules for Targeted Drug Delivery

Another emerging nanotechnology tool is the use of nanocapsules for targeted delivery of detoxifying drugs directly to tissues affected by graphene accumulation. These nanocapsules can be loaded with antioxidant drugs or chelating agents and are designed to recognize and bind to graphene nanoparticles in tissues. Once bound, they release their therapeutic content in a localized manner, reducing the risk of systemic side effects.

Recent studies in Advanced Drug Delivery Reviews have shown that nanocapsules can enhance treatment efficacy by enabling targeted detoxification and shortening patient recovery times. This type of technology could be applied not only to graphene but also to other toxic nanoparticles.

3. Advanced Monitoring Technologies for Nanoparticles

To manage nanoparticles in the body, it is crucial to monitor their presence and accumulation. Advanced monitoring technologies are rapidly evolving, providing increasingly precise and non-invasive tools for detecting graphene in biological tissues.

Graphene Biosensors for Real-Time Detection

An exciting development in advanced diagnostics is the use of graphene-based biosensors to monitor nanoparticle levels in real-time. These sensors, which rely on graphene's electrical conductivity, are highly sensitive and can detect trace amounts of nanoparticles in the blood or bodily fluids. This type of monitoring could enable doctors to identify graphene accumulation early, preventing long-term damage.

A study published in ACS Nano highlighted how graphene biosensors can detect changes in biomarkers linked to inflammation or cell damage induced by nanoparticles. These sensors could be integrated into wearable devices or diagnostic tools, providing continuous assessments of a patient's health status.

Imaging Techniques for Nanoparticle Detection

The use of advanced imaging techniques, such as optical coherence tomography (OCT) or nuclear magnetic resonance (NMR), may allow doctors to directly observe the accumulation of nanoparticles in tissues. These techniques are already used in clinical settings for diagnosing other diseases, and research is exploring how to adapt them for monitoring graphene nanoparticles.

Raman spectroscopy, previously discussed in earlier chapters, remains one of the most promising techniques for precise graphene detection at the cellular level. By combining these imaging techniques with advanced diagnostic tools, it will be possible to obtain a comprehensive and precise evaluation of graphene exposure and accumulation levels in the body.

4. Future Prospects in Nanoparticle Management

The future of nanoparticle management, including graphene, is extremely promising. The continued evolution of medical and pharmacological technologies offers new possibilities for preventing, treating, and detoxifying the body from the potentially harmful effects of nanoparticles.

Personalization of Therapies

One of the most important directions in research is the **personalization of therapies**, developing tailored treatments based on the unique characteristics of each individual. Future drugs and nanotechnologies will be designed to adapt to the genetic profile and specific needs of the patient, allowing for more effective and safer detoxification.

Targeted graphene therapies could vary from person to person, depending on their exposure, metabolism, and ability to eliminate nanoparticles. This personalized approach could greatly improve treatment efficacy while reducing the risk of complications.

Collaborations between Industry and Research

Collaborations between nanotechnology companies and medical researchers are accelerating the development of safe and effective solutions for treating graphene and other nanoparticles. As knowledge advances, it is expected that therapies and monitoring devices will become more accessible, improving public health and reducing the risks of exposure to potentially harmful nanoparticles.

New Safety Protocols

One of the outcomes of these collaborations is the development of new safety protocols for the use of graphene in both industrial and biomedical settings. These protocols include guidelines for handling and exposure to nanoparticles, as well as the use of personal protective equipment and continuous exposure assessments in workplaces. The **World Health Organization (WHO)** and other international institutions are developing stricter standards to ensure that workers exposed to graphene are protected from long-term risks.

Integration of Innovations in Clinical Settings

As research progresses and collaborations between scientists and industries grow, an important direction is the **integration of new graphene-based technologies** into clinical settings. Wearable devices with graphene-based biosensors, nanocapsules for targeted drug delivery, and advanced imaging techniques to monitor nanoparticle accumulation are already being tested in various clinical studies.

These innovations offer non-invasive monitoring capabilities, enabling early diagnosis and personalized treatment for patients exposed to graphene. Clinics may soon have tools capable of continuously monitoring biomarkers in the blood, allowing doctors to quickly assess the need for detoxification or preventive measures.

New Combined Therapies

With the advent of new technologies, research is also exploring **combined therapies** that leverage nanotechnologies and advanced drugs to more effectively treat graphene nanoparticles. Some experimental therapies combine the use of **chelating agents**, which bind and neutralize nanoparticles, with **photothermal therapies**, which use heat generated by the nanoparticles themselves to destroy them or facilitate their degradation.

A study published in Advanced Materials showed promising results in combining these techniques, improving treatment efficacy and reducing side effects. These combined therapies could be particularly useful for people with long-term graphene exposure, ensuring a more comprehensive management of the risk.

Conclusion

The future of nanoparticle management, especially graphene, holds tremendous promise. With ongoing advancements in drug development, nanotechnologies, and monitoring tools, it is likely that new, safer, and more effective methods for detoxifying the body from nanoparticles will emerge. Personalized therapies, combined with innovative monitoring and treatment technologies, will play a crucial role in minimizing the risks associated with graphene exposure, paving the way for safer industrial and medical applications.

In the final chapter, we will summarize the key takeaways from the book and provide actionable steps to help readers apply the insights and strategies shared throughout to protect their health and well-being in an increasingly nanoparticle-filled world.

Final Reflections

This chapter concludes our comprehensive guide on the impact of graphene on the human body, and the natural and technological strategies available for managing its presence. Throughout the book, we've explored how graphene, while heralded for its groundbreaking applications in various fields, poses certain risks when it comes to its accumulation in the body. We have also discussed innovative ways to monitor, detoxify, and protect ourselves from the potential long-term health effects of exposure to this material.

The primary goal has been to provide practical and scientifically supported advice for those concerned about graphene exposure. By incorporating natural detoxification methods, monitoring tools, and emerging technologies, readers are empowered to take proactive steps in safeguarding their health.

It's essential to remain informed about the ongoing research and developments regarding graphene. As technology advances and more is learned about the behavior of nanoparticles in the human body, new and more effective solutions will emerge. By staying educated and adopting a proactive approach, individuals can improve their overall well-being and reduce the potential risks associated with living in an increasingly technologically advanced world.

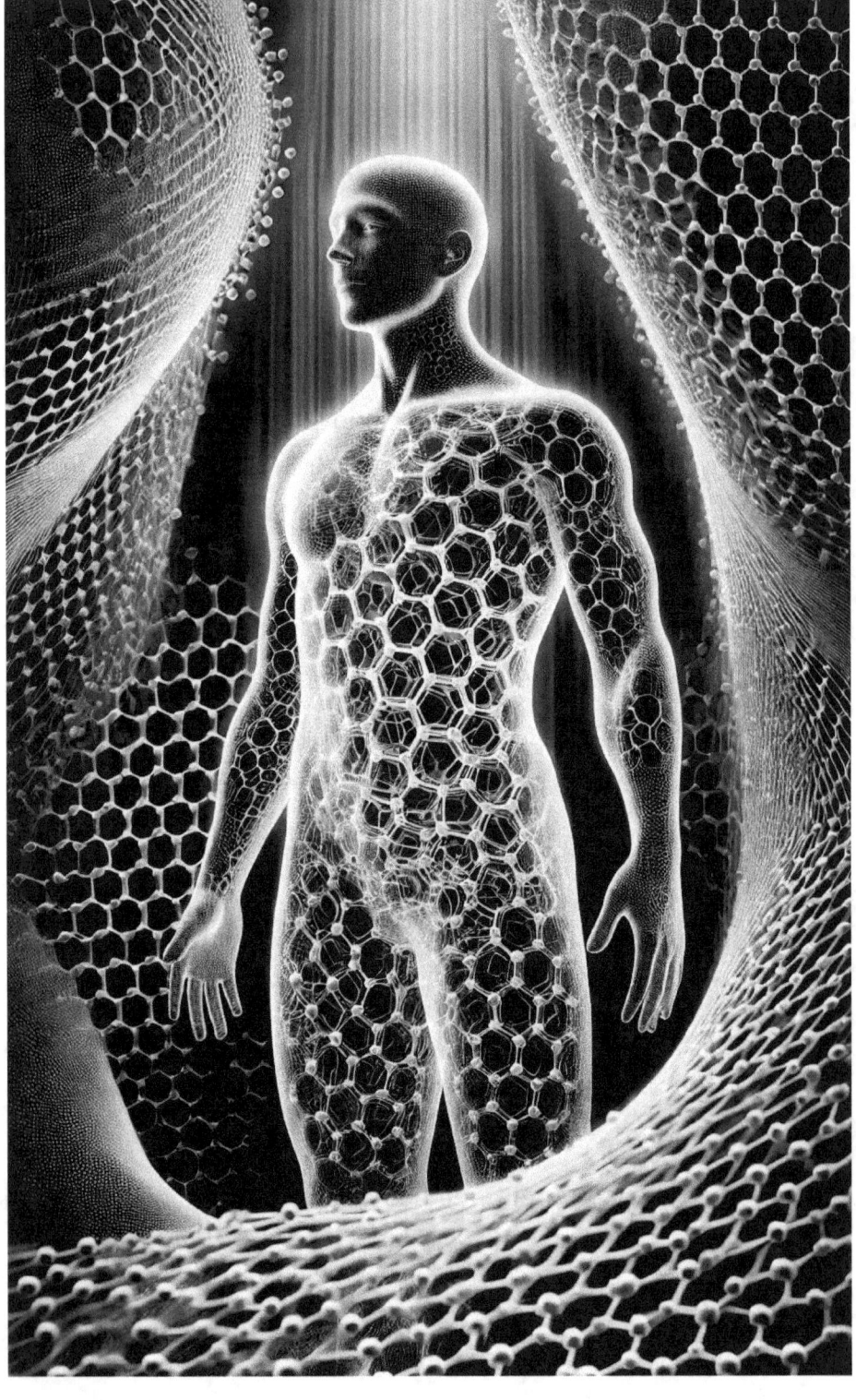

Copyright © 2024 Dr. Adrian Selby. All rights reserved.

This book and its contents are protected by copyright laws and international treaties.

No part of this publication may be reproduced, distributed, translated, stored in a retrieval system, or transmitted in any form or by any means, electronic or mechanical, including photocopies, recordings, or other methods, without the prior written consent of the author or copyright holder, except as provided by law.

Any violation will be subject to legal action.

The quotes contained in this book are attributed to their respective authors when known. In cases of fictitious attributions, they are created solely for narrative purposes and do not imply any relation to real individuals.

Year of publication: 2024

Disclaimer

The information and strategies presented in this book are the result of thorough research and natural practices, but they should not be interpreted as medical diagnoses or cures for any condition. Every individual is unique, and responses to detox programs, dietary changes, or suggested remedies may vary.

The author and publisher do not guarantee the effectiveness or safety of the methods described for all readers, as results may depend on individual factors, including pre-existing health conditions, age, and lifestyle.

Please note that some information may not be recognized or approved by the official medical community. This book is not intended to replace treatments or prescriptions provided by licensed healthcare professionals.

We strongly recommend consulting a qualified professional before making significant changes to your diet, routine, or medical treatments.

www.ingramcontent.com/pod-product-compliance
Lightning Source LLC
Chambersburg PA
CBHW071106240526
45469CB00006BD/2344